Yoga With Intention

A Yogic Life Journey from Awareness to Honoring

John E. Cottrell III, Ph.D.

DEDICATION

This book is dedicated to my parents, John and Joyce, who taught me about perseverance and serving others. This book is also dedicated to all my students who have practiced with me in the yoga studios over the years. It is you who have inspired the words in this book. YOU have helped me to grow, to be more aware, and to honor. Thank you to D'ana Baptiste who gave me the space in her yoga studio to grow, to teach, and to express my truth. And a special thank you to Perry Layne of www.PerryLayneProductions.com for taking all the photos for this book.

TABLE OF CONTENTS

THE INTENTION OF THIS BOOK

The intention of this book is to bring yoga into your everyday life. If you're a regular yoga practitioner, you may have frequented your favorite yoga class a few times a week. You sweat, stretch, relax, and generally feel good after your yoga practice. But what do you do in between your yoga classes? Are you practicing yoga on the mat AND off the mat?

This book will help you to bring your yogic journey into a new light. It will help you create a home yoga practice. You can even use some of the yoga techniques "on-the-go." Use the lessons of this book to guide you through challenging obstacles in your life and move toward freedom, alignment, and balance. The messages and yoga sequences will guide you toward a greater connection to self and stimulate change in your life.

The book is divided into five sections. It is a progression; a journey. We begin with Awareness. We take note of how we are in the current moment. Without judgment, we step outside of ourselves and look inward. Examine the person you are in this very moment. It is only from here that we can start our journey forward. Next, we will begin to Release the parts of self that do not serve us. You may be holding onto stories, beliefs, or emotions that seem irrelevant to who you want to be. The next section takes us on a journey of Growth and Opening. We will discover new parts of ourselves. We will be able to allow our Truth to shine through. Self Care is the next section of this book. This is a time for self-reflection and nurturing. In order for our Truth to emerge and grow, we must do our best to take care of ourselves in a loving, kind, and healthy way. Now that you have come to this new Awareness of Self, it is time to Honor Yourself. Sit back and reflect on the power, strength, and balance, that you truly possess.

Although designed as a progressive journey, you can also use this book as a reference manual, tool, or guide. It is written so that when you have a spare moment in your day, you can open the book to any point, read the life lesson, and practice the short yoga sequence or pose.

The first yoga lesson will not involve any yoga postures. It will simply be a breath practice that helps you to discover relaxation, mindfulness, release, and awareness. Breath is considered the foundation of any yoga practice, so this is a good place to start. What is wonderful about this particular yoga practice is that you can do it anytime and anywhere. Think of it as a quick remedy to ailments that can strike us at anytime during our daily lives. Let's get started....

1.
AWARENESS

"If you want to conquer the anxiety of life, live in the moment, live in the breath."
- Amit Ray

This section will focus on becoming more aware of yourself and your current surroundings and situations. Become more mindful.

1. Awareness & Breath
2. Potential
3. Your Life Purpose
4. Reunion

1. Awareness & Breath

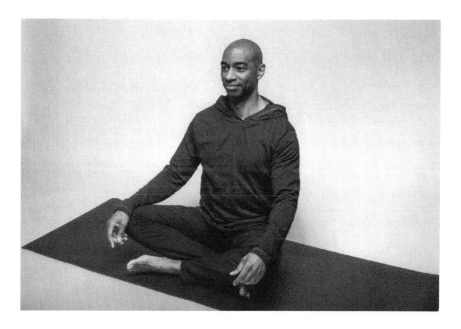

Featured Poses:
Easy Pose (Sukhasana)
Ujjayi Breath

Props:
Soft cushion or folded blanket

The intention of this yoga practice is to bring yourself to greater awareness of self. Sometimes this can be a challenge, especially when we're faced with so many responsibilities and activities in our daily lives. We find that we are continually distracted by life's events that it gives us little time to take care of ourselves. Again, this practice is for YOU so that you can put aside those obligations for a moment and pay attention to your inner needs.

This will be a relatively simple yoga practice. It will focus primarily on your breath. It can also be considered a type of meditation. Breath is the foundation of the yoga practice. It provides a base and structure that allows one to be at peace with self.

Start by sitting comfortably cross-legged on your yoga mat or on the floor. You will be here awhile, so be sure you are very comfortable. Sit on a cushion or blanket to help support your sitting posture. If sitting up on your own is uncomfortable, sit up against a wall. Sit up nice and tall, with your hands and arms fully relaxed. Close your eyes. Take a moment just to settle into your space. Make any adjustments in your body so that you feel as comfortable as possible.

Breath: As you sit in stillness and silence, begin to pay attention to your breathing. You don't have to do anything special or different with your breath at this point. Simply be aware that you are breathing. Inhale and exhale through your nose.

As we focus on the breath, the foundation of the yoga practice, we begin to tune OUT the things going on outside of us and begin to tune IN to the things going on inside of us. Just sit here with breath. Feel your breath. Listen to the sound of your breath. Breathe as if there is nothing else to do. If you cannot hear your breath, begin to breathe a little slower and deeper. Truly begin to experience the flow and feel of your breath.

Let's begin to add more energy to this breathing sensation so that you can be even more aware of the breath inside of you. What follows is a breathing technique that will help you engage the breath and bring more energy to the breath. Right now, you are probably feeling air move through your nostrils. We are going to shift this way of breathing to another that will allow for more intentional breathing. We will engage what is called Ujjayi breath. (Pronounced oo-jah-yee.) This involves using your throat muscles to help move the breath with more effort.

For a moment, open and breathe through your mouth. Pull in breath through the mouth as if you were gasping for air. You may feel a cool sensation hit the back of your throat. Next, breathe out as if you are fogging a mirror. You may feel a warm sensation as the air leaves your mouth. You may even hear a sound, something like the waves of the ocean rushing onto the beach. Now, continue to breathe this way, but with your mouth closed. This is one form of Ujjayi breathing. You may find that you are able to inhale and exhale more slowly with a greater capacity of air. Continue to feel the breath and listen to the sound of the ocean as you exhale.

Breathing this way keeps your attention and focus on yourself. You are breathing with intention. You may discover that you are no longer thinking about your other life obligations. You have simply set them aside for a moment to pay more attention to yourself: awareness. If you are new to this way of breathing, practice this dynamic breath work for 30 seconds to 1 minute. That doesn't sound like a very long time at first, but it's enough time to grow more aware of yourself. It grounds you and you'll feel more connected to yourself. As you continue this breath practice, you may find, over time, that you can do it for a longer period of time.

This is a relatively simple yoga practice and can be done ANYTIME and ANYWHERE. Here's a perfect example. Imagine yourself at work faced with deadlines, to-do lists, and other responsibilities that take up a lot of physical and mental energy. As the work piles up, do you find that "you just can't take it anymore" and need a break? Once you are aware of this thought, stop what you're doing and come back to this practice. Sit in your office chair or better yet, close your office door, shut off the lights, sit on the floor, and take 1-2 minutes to practice your Ujjayi breathing. You may be amazed at the results. Do you feel more relaxed, clear headed, present? Perhaps this little breathing exercise is all you needed to get through the rest of your day. It's sometimes better than grabbing that candy bar or a cup of coffee to get that boost of energy.

Try this exercise if you are having trouble sleeping. Usually, we are distracted by running thoughts in our heads. We may be worrying about tomorrow's assignments or recounting the events of today. With an active mind, it can be difficult to fall asleep. Lie comfortably in your bed. Bring your attention to your breathing. Feel your breath. Listen to the sound of your breath. You'll begin to be more in tuned with your own being which allows those other thoughts to dissipate. Whenever a straying thought emerges, however, simply be aware of the thought, acknowledge it, then return to the breath. Continue this exercise and you may find that the mind and body begin to relax allowing you to go to sleep.

2. Potential

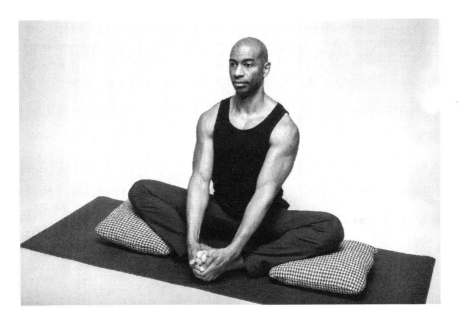

Featured Pose:
Baddha Konasana (Bound Angle Pose)

Props:
Cushion, Pillow, or Blanket, 2 Yoga Blocks

"Open yourself up to your greatest potential." That could certainly be a person's mantra or motivational quote that they have taped to their bathroom mirror! It could also be the intention behind any yoga practice. But what does it really mean? I have often defined yoga to my new yoga students as the practice of finding greater awareness of self by focusing on breath and movement. When you focus on these areas, you find and feel a clarity about yourself that seems to open many doors. You find that you have greater strength, ability, focus, balance, integrity, peace of mind, and the list goes on. Yoga can be the practice that opens the doors to many possibilities. One can start simply and easily to find those inner openings; to discover your own greatest potential.

Bound Angle Pose, also called Cobbler's Pose, named for the Indian cobbler as he sits and builds shoes, is a yoga posture that is essentially a hip opener. The pose can also demonstrate the inner potential one seeks to discover. Start by sitting on the floor and bring the bottoms of your feet together. Draw your heels closer to your pelvis. Your knees will naturally drop down to the side. If your hips are little tight, this is great pose to begin that release. Don't worry if your knees do not touch the floor. They don't need to. In fact, you may also want to place a yoga block (or other object) under each knee if they do not reach the floor. This will allow for greater relaxation in the hips since the knees are literally resting on the blocks, thus easing any tension. Hold onto your toes, ankles or shins so that you are able to sit up tall with an extended spine. (Feel free to practice this pose sitting against a wall. You can also do Supta Baddha Konasana, or Reclining Bound Angle Pose which is done lying on your back.) To find more comfort and ease in this pose, feel free to sit on a yoga block, blanket, or cushion. This naturally raises the hips over the knees in this posture allowing for the hips to open up more.

Once you have established the pose, set your intention. Perhaps you want to be more extroverted or be able to speak your mind more freely and with confidence. Maybe you feel stuck in a rut and want to find a way to move forward; create a change in the old routine. When our minds and bodies are opened, we can see the possibilities; the doors begin to open. Cobbler's Pose can guide you toward feeling more alive, free, and open.

Hold here for 10-15 breaths. Allow the natural release and the opening to occur. If you focus on the exhale, this can assist the release of any tightness in the inner thighs and hips. Further, if your intention is to open yourself up more, then this, too, will happen with the practice of this pose. Remember your initial intention and experience the revealing of your natural potential.

3. Your Life Purpose

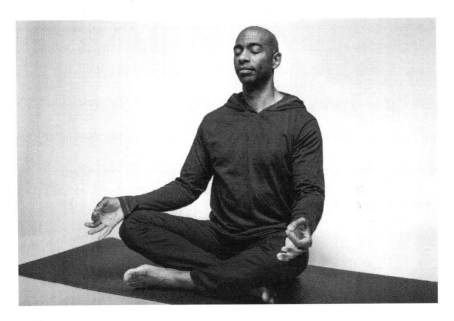

<u>Featured Poses:</u>
Easy Pose (Sukhasana)
Ujjayi Breath

<u>Props:</u> Soft cushion or folded blanket (optional)

In the ancient scripture, The Bhagavad Gita, Krishna speaks of dharma - your life purpose. He tells his student warrior, "...it is better to do your own dharma poorly than to do someone else's well."

This, I believe, is good advice. We can certainly get caught in our lives wishing that it resembled SOMEONE ELSE'S LIFE! "I wish my house was as big as hers." "I like her style. I'm going to dress just like her." "If only I had a job like his." When we find ourselves in these thoughts, we are slowly moving away from our True Authentic Selves. If we take a moment in stillness and silence, we reconnect to that True Self. Know what it is that makes you uniquely You! Discover what it is that you are able to do. Not only what you are ABLE to do, but what you LOVE to do.

What is your Passion? Often, it is this Passion that grows into your Life Purpose - your dharma.

How may times have you gone to a yoga class and the person next to you is more flexible than you, or can hold a pose longer than you, or is wearing a cooler outfit? Yoga is not about comparing or competing. We have the opportunity to share our energies in a community, but the yoga practice is really for YOU. It is your moment, your opportunity to journey deeply within yourself to discover your dharma. Krishna says that your dharma "need not be lofty, but should be something that feels right to you, and something that in one way or another makes a contribution."

Perhaps your passion is working with children, or photography, or cooking, or singing. The list is endless, but tune in and find out what it is that moves you. That talent may end up to be something that is worth sharing with others around you.

In your home practice, simply sit in stillness. Focusing on your breath. Allow the time with self be a personal journey inward to uncover your talents, passions, and life purpose. This is something you can do everyday. The more you move within, the more you discover about yourself. Also, when you return to the yoga studio, continue this inward journey. Don't let the more flexible or finely dressed yogi next to you distract you from your personal work. Return to your breath and unleash your Authentic Self.

4. Reunion

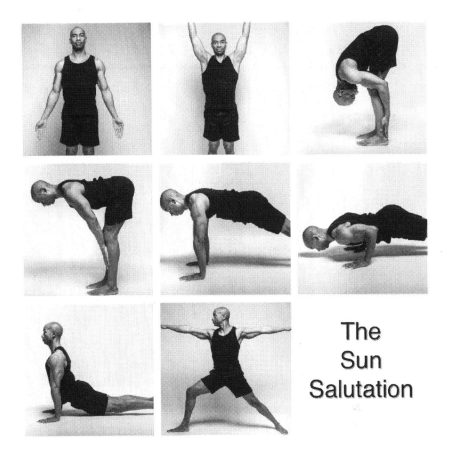

The
Sun
Salutation

Featured Poses:
Sun Salutations (Surya Namaskara)
Easy Pose (Sukhasana)

I've entitled this chapter "Reunion" because it reminds me of the definition of yoga. The Sanskrit word, yoga, literally means "yoke." I have also heard the ancient word interpreted as "joining" or "union." As we practice the asanas (postures) we move and breathe with the intention of joining Mind, Body, and Spirit. The yoga postures are the vehicles that help us to begin that journey.

As a celebration of the yoga practice, I offer to you a home practice that reminds us of the unions we have established in our lives.

Bring to Mind those that are important to you: good friends, family members, classmates, yoga friends, work colleagues, etc. Bring to Mind those that have been great influences in your life. Create vivid pictures of these people in your Mind's eye as you set your intention for your practice. Perhaps you want to thank them or send good intentions their way.

Now it's time for your moving practice. Come to a standing position at the top of your yoga mat: Mountain Pose.

The Sun Salutation (Surya Namaskara: Series A)
Inhale: Extend your arms overhead. Reach for the sky. (Extended Mountain Pose)

Exhale: Fold forward to touch your toes. Bend your knees as you fold in order to protect your back. (Forward Fold)

Inhale: Slide your hands lightly up to your shins and extend your spine until your back is flat. ("Monkey Pose")

Exhale: Plant your hands into the floor and step, walk, or jump back to plank pose. Continue the exhale as you now lower your body to the floor by bending your elbows. Keep your back flat and core engaged. (Chaturanga Dandasana: Four Limbed Staff Pose)

Inhale: Lift your upper body and hips off the floor by pressing your hands into the mat and straightening your arms. You will create a backbend. (Upward Facing Dog)

Exhale: Lift your hips into the air creating an inverted V-shape with your body. Keep your knees slightly bent so that your back stays flat. (Downward Facing Dog)

Inhale: Fill yourself up with breath to prepare your body to move.

Exhale: Jump, step, or walk both feet back up to the top of your mat.

Inhale: Slide your hands lightly up to your shins and extend your spine until your back is flat. ("Monkey Pose")

Exhale: Forward Fold

Inhale: Rise all the way back up to a standing position and extend your arms into the air. (Extended Mountain Pose)

Exhale: Bring your hands to heart-center. (Mountain Pose)

Practice 3-5 Sun Salutations to bring movement to your Body. The complete Sun Salutation offers stretches, backbends, forward folds, strength, stamina, and cleansing to the Body. This physical discipline allows for greater connection to ourselves as well as greater opening, awareness, and deeper connections to others.

After your Sun Salutes, simply sit in a cross-legged posture (Easy Pose) and become more mindful of your breath (Pranayama). Here, sit in stillness having set your intention and moved your body. In stillness, you heighten the work of the Spirit within you. With this raised energy, you truly see your authentic Self and how you share that Self with your outer world. The Spirit within that is allowed to come to the surface through an intentional yoga practice is what your friends and family see: it's your Truth.

So, in celebration of your Yoga, Your Internal Union, and your Union with others, move through this simple practice and be thankful for those people closest to you who see you for who you really are.

2.
RELEASE

"Patience and perseverance have a magical effect before which difficulties disappear and obstacles vanish."
- John Quincy Adams

This section will focus on being aware of the obstacles that we are often faced with. Sometimes those obstacles show up as tensions in the body. The yoga poses described here will help you identify those tensions and begin the journey toward moving past them.

1. Letting Go of What No Longer Serves You
2. Getting Over Obstacles
3. Getting Out of Binds
4. Wring It Out

1. Letting Go of What No Longer Serves You

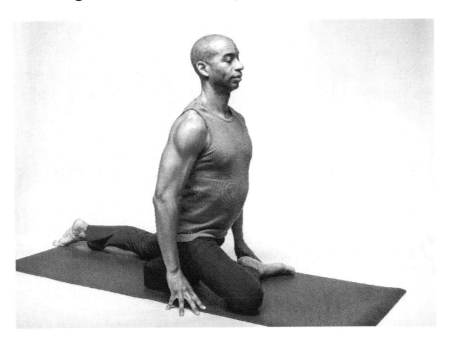

Featured Pose:
Pigeon Pose (Eka Pada Rajakapotasana)

Props:
Block (optional)

As you begin this section of the book and prepare for your yoga practice, bring to mind thoughts, feelings, and beliefs that you hold onto. As you stand in Mountain Pose on your mat, connect to your breath. Gain a greater connection to yourself with full, deep, and complete breaths in and out of your nose.

As you continue to connect to self, again, be aware of the thoughts, feelings and beliefs you hold onto. Are these thoughts and feelings ones you want to guide you through your days? Are the beliefs you have truly your own or do they come from other sources like your parents, teachers, or church? Take a moment with your breath and determine how they influence you and how you walk through your life. Do they serve you well? Do they reflect who you are today? Do they reflect who you want to be? If the answer is "no" to any of these questions, then maybe this is your opportunity to begin releasing the thoughts, feelings, and beliefs that no longer serve you. Begin the process of opening yourself up to new thoughts and beliefs that truly reflect who you are today and/or who you would like to be in the future.

This yoga practice will feature poses that invite release and create an opening for which to generate new thoughts, new feelings, and new beliefs that may better serve you on your life journey.

Begin with a few Sun Salutations to bring warmth to your body. Integrate the following poses and intentions as you invite more opening to your life.

Pigeon Pose allows for the body to experience both resistance and release. As you focus on the thoughts, feelings, and beliefs that may no longer serve you, also be aware of why you still tend to hold onto them. Do they give you a sense of satisfaction, fulfillment, or sense of identity? What would happen if you decided to let go of them?

Let's say, for example, that you are holding on to a notion that you are not talented in a certain area. Ask yourself: "who told you that you were not talented?" Did someone say you could not sing, play baseball, or write poetry? Because of these external opinions, have you limited your singing, ball playing, or writing? If you feel that you truly hold a talent or strength in a certain area, give yourself the permission to express it. Move through the resistance of external influences and open yourself to your greatest potential.

In Pigeon Pose, be mindful of the sensation in your outer hips and thighs as you hold this pose. If you feel tightness or even discomfort, this may represent resistance. As you continue to breathe with ease (slowly in and slowly out) you might find yourself more comfortable in the pose, even moving deeper into the posture. This is you giving way to the resistance, the external influence, and rising into your own. Stay here for at least 10 breaths. Perform the same pose on the other side.

If this pose is too stressful on your knees, here is an alternative way to experience a similar stretch. Lie flat on your back, knees bent with your feet flat on the floor. Cross your right ankle over your left knee (actually just below the knee). With your right hand, gently push the right knee away from you. You may experience sensation in your right glute as a nice stretch. This will also open the hip. To add more sensation to this pose, lift your left foot and draw that knee toward your chest. Continue to gently push the right knee away from you. Hold for at least 10 breaths and repeat the sequence on the other side.

Complete your practice by lying in Savasana for 3 to 5 minutes. Use this restorative posture to continue the intention of tension release.

Our hips tend to hold a lot of emotional stress and tension. Use this practice to help find emotional relief and relaxation.

2. Getting Over Obstacles

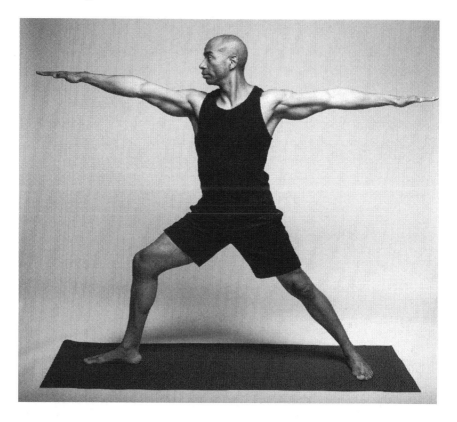

<u>Featured Poses:</u>
Transition from Downward Facing Dog (Adho Mukha Svanasana) to
Warrior I & II (Virabhadrasana I & II)

<u>Props:</u>
Block

As you prepare for this home yoga practice, take a moment to think
about the things in your life that seem to hold you back from moving
forward. It can be anything from a lack of money, minor symptoms of
depression, or a boss that is reluctant to give you a raise. Whatever it is,
we often see these things as obstacles in our lives. What do you do in
response to these obstacles? Do you remain stuck with no vision of
advancement? Do you continue to beat the wall, but feel like you're not

making any progress? Do you become angry, frustrated, disillusioned, or feel betrayed?

What if you could see yourself moving past these obstacles? Recall the strengths that you have (organized, intelligent, fast learner, excellent chef, etc.) It is these same strengths, talents, and traits that will allow you to move past, through, and around these obstacles.

Begin in Mountain Pose. As you begin here, take a moment to recall the calming feeling of your breath. Be aware of the unguarded nature of the breath. Experience how it continues to flow without much effort. Allow this experience of breath to guide you through your yoga practice today.

Start your flow with three Sun Salutations to warm the body. As you move, call to mind the obstacles with which you are currently dealing. As breath guides you through these few Sun Salutations, experience the opening quality of the breath. The breath will be your tool to break down the walls that might hold you back from advancing forward on your life journey. Each pose in the Sun Salutation has a definite intention of opening you. Give yourself the same permission to open yourself up, to move through your current challenges, and press forward.

Now, let's add an obstacle to your sequence: the yoga block. Place the block in the middle of your mat, then come to a Downward Facing Dog position. Imagine the block as that obstacle you've been dealing with. In this inverted posture, you should be able to see the block. As you inhale, extend your right leg into the air. Exhale, engage your core, shift your body forward, bend your knee, and step OVER the block. (Did you make it?) Did you kick the block, go around it, hit it, or clear it? Just NOTICE what happens as you get your foot to the top of your mat. (Did you react?) Did you chastise yourself for hitting the block? Celebrate that you got over it? Just be aware of your emotional reaction to the obstacle. Finish the flow by rising to Warrior I. Now, bring your hands down to the mat to frame your right foot and step your LEFT foot over the block bringing both feet to the top of your mat into Forward Fold. Rise to Extended Mountain Pose and finish by placing your hands at heart-center.

Continue with the Sun Salutation knowing that you will have to JUMP over the block (or step over it) when you transition your feet to the back of your mat. Once again, notice how it felt to get OVER THE OBSTABCLE. When you arrive at Downward Facing Dog, proceed with extending your left leg into the air and follow the same flow.

When you've completed this round, challenge yourself by moving the block slightly FORWARD. Try the sequence again. All the while, continue to notice your thoughts and emotions as you move through this sequence.

Although this is just a yoga sequence with a block, it can certainly be a metaphor as to how we deal with obstacles in our everyday lives off the yoga mat. Sometimes we may celebrate when we achieve our goals and break through barriers. Other times we may become frustrated or upset if we make mistakes or "can't" get past the seemingly impossible ordeal. Notice these reactions, then return to the calming breath. Even in times of distress COME BACK TO YOUR BREATH. It can be the guiding force that allows you to move forward. Breath can be the key to persistence and eventual success.

3. Getting Out of Binds

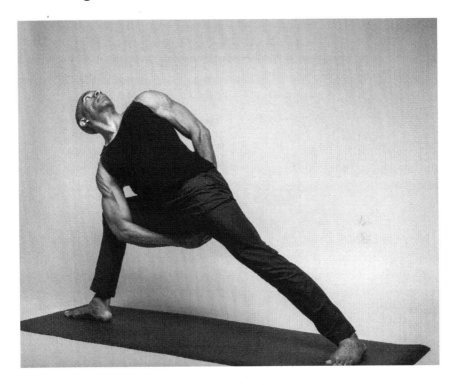

Featured Poses:
Bound Extended Side Angle Pose (Baddha Utthita Parsvakonasana)

Props:
Yoga Strap or Hand Towel

Ever find yourself in a bind? You know, you have to get the kids to soccer practice AND you have to be at an important meeting at the same time. Or you've been asked to speak at a benefit event on a particular evening AND you have tickets to see your favorite music group in concert the same night. Or even more simply, you don't know which outfit to wear one morning. These may not seem like very significant binds to be in. There are certainly more emotional and/or physical binds that we can find ourselves in: should I really be in this relationship? which college should I attend? do I get surgery on my knee or live with the pain? The question becomes....how do you get yourself

OUT of these binds?

Sometimes we can feel overwhelmed when we are faced with such a question, especially when the decision appears to be quite confusing or nearly impossible to make. You may think, "how will this affect me and my life journey?" "How will my decision affect other people?" Before you have to make the decision, why not just take a moment, pause, and take a few breaths. A simple clearing of the mind may help your decision making to get out of the bind.

This yoga practice gives us insight into how we often put ourselves into our own binds, but it also shows how we have the strength and aptitude to get ourselves out of those binds.

Start by standing in a Warrior II Pose with your right foot forward on your yoga mat. Your torso will be long and tall, perpendicular to the floor. Here you may set your intention. Take a few deep breaths to clear your mind. From here, slowly extend you right hand and arm forward out over your right thigh. This will create an angle in the torso, about 45 degrees. Once you can no longer extend your arm forward creating this angle in the upper body, rotate your arms so your left arm is extending upward toward the ceiling and your right arm is extending down toward the floor. (Be sure your torso remains open to the side of the room rather than facing down toward the floor.)

Here is where you will create the bind in the pose. Bring your left arm down behind you. See if you can wrap it around your waist or have your hand up close to your right hip rather than along your buttocks. Next, reach your right arm underneath your right thigh. Bend that arm to reach up for your left set of fingers. (If you are unable to bring your two hands together behind you in this bind, using a prop like a towel or strap may help you get into this pose.) See if you can keep your right arm along your hamstring rather than directly between your legs.

As you are able, continue extending your spine so that the crown of your head is pointing directly forward just as your right knee is pointing directly forward. Your heart and torso will still be open to the side of the room. Hold this posture for 5-10 breaths. Feel the pressure this creates in your legs, arms, back, and hips. Allow this to mimic the binds that we sometimes find ourselves in. Squeeze a little tighter to experience how challenging some of those life binds can be. After your series of breaths, slowly begin to move out of the pose....out of the bind. Take your time, so you can fully experience the sensation of release. Feel how the body, mind, and breath feel free as you have now moved out of the bind. Make your way back up to the Warrior II Pose. Come to a full standing posture (Mountain Pose) before you do the other side.

It is common for us to face situations in our lives where we will feel overwhelmed with complicated decision making. We worry about the outcome and how it might affect other people like our partners, co-workers, children, and friends. Be mindful that whatever decision that is made, it has been made with honesty, a sense of honor and compassion, and with intention.

4. Wring It Out

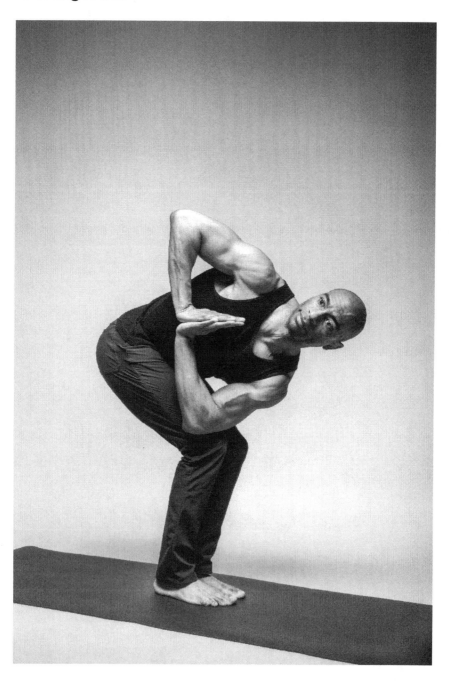

Featured Poses:
Twisted Chair Pose (Parivritta Utkatasana)

Props:
Block (optional)

Practicing poses like Pigeon Pose and Standing Forward Fold can help you to release some of the tensions that are stored in your body. Here is a great practice that will help you to feel cleansed of those uncomfortable sensations in your body.

This yoga posture can provide a sense of healing and detoxification. Whenever I instruct a twisting pose in a yoga class, I have the students imagine that they are a wet sponge ready to be wrung out. When a sponge is wet, it is typically heavy - saturated with a substance that is ready to move out. When one wrings out a sponge, all the water is released, leaving it light and virtually empty - ready to absorb new content. Hold onto this image as you practice this next pose.

Start your practice in Mountain Pose with your hands at your Heart Center to set your intention. Perhaps you have been sitting heavy with thoughts, worries, aches, pains, and concern that you are ready to release. Think of those ideas and sensations as the water in the saturated sponge.

Inhale to extend your arms overhead. Exhale and sit back into Chair Pose. Keep your arms extended alongside your ears. Sit back as if you are sitting in an imaginary chair. Shift your weight back slightly so the weight is in the heels of your feet. (You should be able to lift or tap your toes easily.) Also, your knees will begin to move to be more aligned over your ankles. (This will also take pressure off the knees and shins.) Next, bring your hands to Heart Center.

With the next few breaths, remain in this pose to further elongate the spine. With each exhale, draw your belly button up toward your spine engaging the Abdominal Lock. When you are ready, exhale and begin a slow twist to the right. You want to be sure to make this a full abdominal twist to simulate wringing out the sponge. Here are some things you can be aware of while moving deeply into the pose:

1) Be sure your feet are still firm on the floor with an even weight distribution between them. Notice if you have rolled to the inner or outer parts of your feet when you twist.

2) Look down at your knees. Be certain that your knees are still aligned with one another. If you are twisting to the right and your left knee shifts forward, then you have moved out of alignment and have decreased the fullest twist possible. (Feel free to use a Yoga Block between your thighs to help stabilize your feet and knees.) If your knees remain aligned, this also means your hips will remain aligned ensuring a full twist rather than a simple turning of your body to the right.

3) Move slowly. There is no need to wring out the sponge all at once. Use several breaths to reach your fullest depth of the pose. Inhale to continue lengthening through your spine and twist a little bit more when you exhale. (Remember to draw your navel in toward your spine.) Keep moving like this until you have reached a full twist. Hold the pose for an additional 5 breaths.

Return to Chair Pose then Mountain Pose. As you unwind from this twist, imagine the wet sponge is now free of it's contents feeling light and newly absorbent. Repeat the pose on the other side.

It is easy for us to walk through our days, weeks, even months feeling heavy with pressure and stress. We become saturated with these feelings and can no longer absorb any more leading to feeling overwhelmed and burned out. Practice this twisted pose to relieve yourself of these burdensome circumstances.

3.
GROWTH & OPENING

"Without continual growth and progress, such words as improvement, achievement, and success have no meaning." - Benjamin Franklin

This section will focus on the progress that you have made so far in becoming more mindful of the obstacles and challenges in your life and now growing from these experiences. You will experience yoga poses that will help you to develop a stronger sense of self. You will feel more confident, secure, and successful in yourself and the activities you take on in life.

1. Open Your Heart
2. Bring New Life to Your Routine
3. Potential
4. Do Your Best
5. Be Victorious

1. Open Your Heart

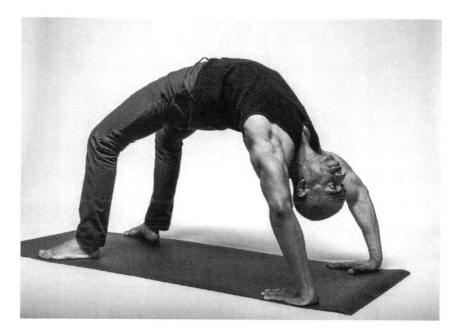

Featured Pose:
Urdhva Dhanurasana (Upward Facing Bow Pose)

Backbends in yoga are considered heart openers. On a day-to-day basis, we can find our body postures in a constant state of "forward folds." Think about it: sitting down at a desk hunched over a computer, cycling, weeding the garden, or other body positions like this are all "heart closers." Doing heart opening postures not only can improve your posture, but they can have an emotional benefit as well.

Think for a moment about your life experiences in the recent past. Have you ever felt sad or depressed? just got dumped by your significant other? got ripped off on a financial deal? All of these situations can bring a sense of hurt, violation, or betrayal. All of these can be very challenging emotional situations to manage. After experiencing such events, it may be difficult to trust; your heart may even feel broken. These may create a "closing of the heart." As a means to help mend your heart from that sense of betrayal, yoga backbends may help you to re-open your heart and teach you to trust again.

This home practice will describe Urdhva Dhanurasana (which literally translates to upward facing bow). This pose is commonly called Wheel Pose; it is a full backbend. If you are new to this pose, a Bridge Pose is a good alternative.

Start by lying on your yoga mat on your back. Bend your knees so your feet are flat on the floor. Be sure your heels are relatively close to your back side and your knees and feet are hip distance apart. This will give you a strong foundation when you rise into the backbend. This sense of connection to the earth is actually a good starting point for the mending heart. You want to feel safe and secure before you move forward in being able to trust again.

Next, place your hands up by your shoulders. Your fingertips should be pointing toward your shoulders with your hands pressing firmly into the floor. To help get the hands secure on the mat, squeeze your elbows together toward your head. It is important to have your fingertips point TOWARD your shoulders rather than have your hands and finders UNDER your shoulders. If your hands are underneath your shoulders, you will not have the best alignment and strength to lift yourself up into the backbend. With your fingertips pointing toward your shoulders, your elbows will be directly over your wrists creating a right angle. This will give you better leverage to rise into your posture. Again, you want to have a strong foundation before you rise into this dynamic pose.

Your core body must also feel secure before rising into the Wheel Pose. As you lie on your back, begin an intentional breathing practice. When you inhale, arch your back. Your bottom will remain on the floor while your low back lifts away from the floor. When you exhale, strongly press your low back into the yoga mat. Your navel will move closer to your spine and your pelvis will naturally tilt to engage your low abdominal muscles. Hold this posture as you continue breathing. With each exhale, continue to tighten your lower abdominals as a means to support your back when you eventually rise into your backbend. Engaging your core body is another practice of finding strength within yourself when you are faced with challenging life obstacles.

When you feel ready (perhaps after 5-10 breaths) lift your hips toward the sky. You are now in a modified Bridge Pose. Even as you lift your hips toward the ceiling, continue to engage your core body as if you were still lying flat on your mat with your lower back pressed into the earth. This will keep your lower back open and spacious so you don't experience binding or pinching in your lower back muscles and spine. Again, if you are new to this style of pose, feel free to remain here for the rest of your practice.

In this modified posture, check in with your body to be sure your feet are still planting firmly into the floor as well as your hands. When you are ready, press your hands deeply into the ground in order to lift your head off the floor. Let the very top of your head rest lightly on the mat. This is another variation on the pose. On your next exhale, press your hands firmly into the mat so you can lift entirely off the floor. You are now in a full backbend. Hold for at least 5 breaths and up to 10. Root your feet and hands firmly into the earth: feel grounded and connected. Allow your heart to expand and open. Be mindful of all the love that IS in the world and absorb that gift: you truly deserve it.

When you are ready to come down, tuck your chin in toward your neck. Lower yourself slowly so that you land softly on the back of your shoulders. Proceed to come all the way down to the floor and lie in Savasana for at least 20 breaths. As you are in your relaxation posture, think about ways you can continue filling your heart with love, gratitude, and appreciation.

2. Bring New Life to Your Routine

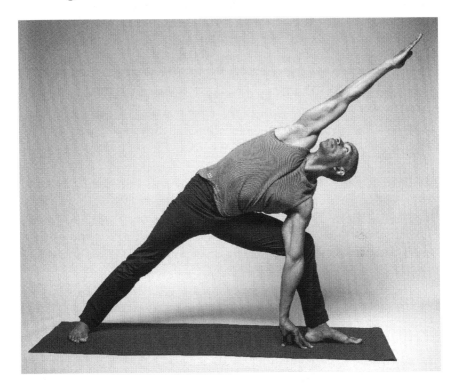

<u>Featured Pose:</u>
Utthita Parsvakonasana (Extended Side Angle Pose, Variations)

Are you stuck in a rut? Do you do the same thing day in and day out? What's that old saying..."variety is the spice of life?" Well, how about adding a little spice in YOUR life! Sometimes our lives can seem routine, rote, and even boring at times. So, is it possible to take that same (boring) routine and make it a whole new experience? How can you bring life, energy, and SPICE to your life journey?

Let's begin on the yoga mat. Even the routine on the yoga mat can get a little rote; particularly the Sun Salutation. It is a basic flow that can feel pretty repetitive at times. You can spice up the flow, however, by focusing on different aspects of the sequence: the pace of your movement, the depth of your poses, the intensity of your breath. All of these (and more) can bring new life to your routine.

Let's take a particular yoga pose Extended Side Angle Pose (Utthita Parsvakonasana) and bring new life to this posture. Start by coming to a Warrior II pose with your right foot in front (leg bent at 90 degrees) and your (straight) left leg in back. Be sure your hips are aligned and can experience the hip opening effect of the posture. Your upper body should be nice and tall as if you were standing in Mountain Pose. To move into Extended Side Angle Pose, reach and move your right arm forward out over your knee and foot. This will put your torso at about a 45 degree angle.

For the first version of this pose, simply place your right hand on your thigh while you extend your left hand toward the ceiling. In this modified version of the pose, you can really focus on proper alignment of the hips and keeping your heart open to the side of the room without feeling like your heart/chest is falling down toward the floor. Remain here for at least 5 breaths.

Now, to add some variety to the pose, begin to take it deeper by placing your right forearm on your thigh. This may intensify the pose. Because it may feel more intense, be sure to keep your focus on the breath, the depth of the new variation of the pose, and stay in tuned with your alignment. Be mindful of this new sensation. Remain here for another 5 breaths.

To complete this side, now take your right hand and place it on the floor next to your right foot. This, too, should change the sensation of the pose. Feel the extended stretch as you have now moved deeper into this angled hip opening pose. Remain here for 5 breaths. The pose itself, has not changed. It is still Extended Side Angle Pose, but YOU have the ability to change the intensity of the pose. Going deeper, for example, may provide more opening and release for tight inner thighs. Going lighter (with your hand on your thigh) may help you with alignment, balance and focus. Repeat this series on your left side.

If you'd like, repeat this pose on both sides again. This time choose new variations: try placing your hand on the outside of your foot. How about binding the pose? (With right foot forward, your right arm will reach underneath your right leg and up towards your right hip. Drop your left arm down behind you and see if you can clasp fingers.)

Imagine doing the same thing with other routines in your life. YOU can add variety and change to your life experience to bring more intensity or lightness - whatever your heart and soul are needing at the moment. Here are some very simple examples: take a different driving route to work; don't put cream and sugar in your morning coffee one day; re-arrange the furniture in your bedroom; order something new at your favorite restaurant; attend a yoga class taught by a different instructor.

3. Potential

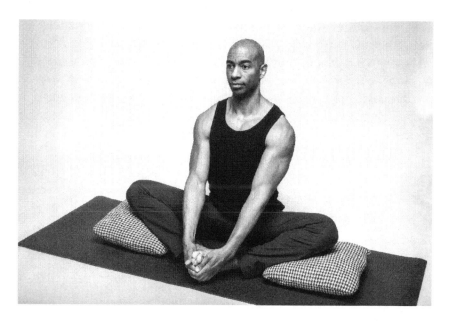

Featured Pose:
Baddha Konasana (Bound Angle Pose)

Props:
Two Blocks or Cushions (optional)

"Open yourself up to your greatest potential." That could certainly be a person's mantra or motivational quote that they have taped to their bathroom mirror! It could also be the intention behind any yoga practice. But what does it really mean? I have often defined yoga to my new yoga students as the practice of finding greater awareness of self by focusing on breath and movement. When you focus on these areas, you find and feel a clarity about yourself that seems to open many doors. You find that you have greater strength, ability, focus, balance, integrity, peace of mind, and the list goes on. Yoga can be the practice that opens the doors to many possibilities. One can start simply and easily to find those inner openings; to discover your own greatest potential.

Bound Angle Pose, also called Cobbler's Pose, named for the Indian cobbler as he sits and builds shoes, is essentially a hip opener, but can also demonstrate that inner potential one seeks to discover. Start by sitting on the floor and bring the bottoms of your feet together. Draw your heels closer to your pelvis. Your knees will naturally drop down to the side. Don't worry if your knees do not touch the floor. They don't need to. If your hips are little tight, this is great pose to begin that release. Hold onto your toes, ankles or shins so that you are able to sit up tall with an extended spine. (Feel free to practice this pose sitting against a wall. You can also do Supta Baddha Konasana, or Reclining Bound Angle Pose which is done lying on your back.)

Once you have established the pose, set your intention. Perhaps you want to be more extroverted or be able to speak your mind more freely and with confidence. Maybe you feel stuck in a rut and want to find a way to move forward; create a change in the old routine. When our minds and bodies are opened, we can see the possibilities; the doors begin to open. Cobbler's Pose can guide you toward feeling more alive, free, and open.

Hold here for 10-15 breaths. Allow the natural release and the opening to occur. If you focus on the exhale, this can assist the release of any tightness in the inner thighs and hips. Remember, it's not necessary to touch the floor with your knees. In fact, use two yoga blocks as support for your knees if they are raised away from the floor. When your knees/legs rest on the blocks, they will feel more relaxed; the muscles of the inner thighs and hips will ease and loosen. If your legs hover over the floor without the use of the blocks, this may create a sense of resistance, a pull, or a struggle for the leg and hip muscles to deal with. Such resistance may inhibit the possibility of fluidly opening. If your intention is to open your mind up more, then this, too, will happen with the practice of this pose. Allow your mind and body to easily and fluidly open without resistance to reach your full potential.

4. Do Your Best

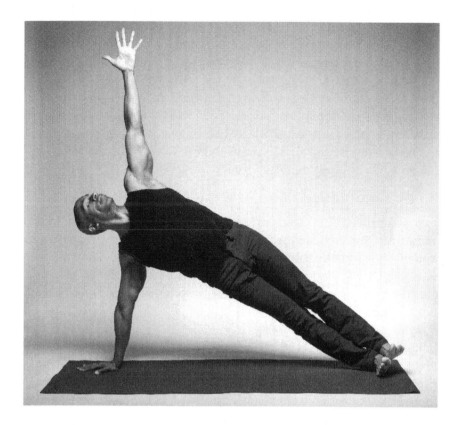

Featured Pose:
Vasisthasana (Side Plank Pose)

Props:
Blanket or towel (optional)

I've been doing some more reading about some common yoga poses and came across an interesting story about Side Plank Pose. But before I get to that, I want to mention that when I work with students individually or with students in a group yoga class, I'm not too concerned if the poses they are performing are absolutely perfect. I just invite my students to do their very best. I offer cues for better alignment and breath flow so that the student feels comfortable in their yoga postures. Also, I provide modifications and variations of poses that support the body.

Recently, I have been working with several students who are new to the yoga practice. One of their main concerns is if they are doing it "right" so they don't look "stupid." I encourage them to not worry too much about "doing it right." The yoga postures are new to them, so it may be challenging at first. I provide plenty of visual and audio cues to help them through the process. The idea is for them to learn the basic concepts to get a general feeling of some of the poses and to experience the yoga breath. Modifications are also demonstrated to help guide them into poses. If they continue to practice yoga, they will see a natural improvement. Again, all I ask is that they do their best. Put in the effort and the time, and they will experience the wonderful benefits of yoga.

The pose I was reading about was Side Plank Pose. In Sanskrit, the language of yoga, it is Vasisthasana (vah-sish-TAHS-anna). Vasistha literally means "most excellent, best, or richest." I thought it would be the perfect pose to write about if you're new to the yoga practice. Yoga can be challenging. It takes energy, strength, effort, and time. But when done with intention and you do your very best, you will have a successful yoga practice.

Even if you're a seasoned practitioner and you're dealing with things in your life right now where you don't feel quite as adequate or confident in yourself as you'd like, consider practicing Vasisthasana. Perhaps you're working on a project at work and you're having trouble getting motivated or you're stuck. Or maybe you made a mistake while answering a question at school. Or maybe you didn't "feel like your normal self" around your family or friends. All of these scenarios can make you feel a little down about yourself. Remember, though, that we ALL make mistakes, get stuck, or say things we do not intend. Overall, we are still trying to do our very best on this life journey. Remind yourself of that as you practice Side Plank Pose.

Start in Plank Pose. It is basically the top of a push-up. You may also place your knees on the floor as a modification if you feel you do not have the upper body strength for this pose. Plank is a very dynamic posture and can add great upper body and core strength. Be sure to feel an energetic movement forward through the crown of your head. At the same time, feel an energetic movement through the heels of your feet.

43

It should feel like you are extending in opposite directions. Further, be sure to engage your core by drawing your navel up toward your spine on an exhale. Maintain this bodily sensation as you move into Side Plank.

Keep your right hand on the yoga mat as you open your body sideways. Your left leg will be stacked on top of the right and your left hand will be reaching up to the ceiling. (Modify the pose by placing your right knee on the floor directly under your hip to help support this posture. For further support, place a blanket or towel under your knee to project your joints.) In this posture, feel free to stack your feet (the inner edges of your feet will touch), or stagger your feet so one is in front of the other for greater stability.

So that there isn't too much pressure in your wrist and shoulder, gently push your pelvis forward on an exhale and lift your left hip up toward the ceiling. You will create a bit of a bend in the body that will send energy and strength down the legs and core body so that the arm does not take the load of this pose. If you are able, left your left leg up so it is parallel with the floor. Keep extending that leg and foot toward the wall to maintain energy in the leg. Also, feel the right inner thigh lift up toward the left inner thigh. This, too, provides great stability for the pose. In this "star" shape, you are now in Vasisthasana - the most excellent and best pose! Hold for 5 slow breaths, return to plank, then proceed to the other side.

While in Side Plank Pose, you will feel the entire body shine; it is fully engage from head to toe. The energy you experience while performing this posture can help you in everyday life situations. When you're down, confused, lacking self confidence, or you don't feel motivated, re-energize your body, mind and spirit with this excellent posture.

5. Be Victorious

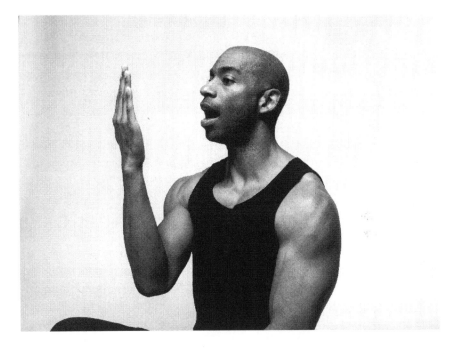

Featured Pose:
Sukhasana (Easy Pose) & Ujjayi Pranayama (Victorious Breath)

The foundation of any yoga practice is the breath. It is the fundamental element that helps the practitioner become more aware of the Self. It allows the yogi to move deeper into themselves. When one is able to sit in stillness with their breath, a sense of calm and peace can be achieved.

The act of breathing is an involuntary operation: we don't have to think about breathing in and out....it just happens. In the yoga practice, however, we breathe with intention and effort. Again, this allows for a greater connection to Self. When we pay attention to the flow of breath, it is difficult to think about anything else. You become centered, present, and balanced just by focusing on the inhales and exhales.

Ujjayi Breath is a style of breathing that is typically done during the yoga practice that keeps the practitioner aware and present. The word ujjayi means "victorious breath" and in this home practice, we will focus on being more victorious in and with ourselves. Below is a description of one way you can practice the Ujjayi Breath or Victorious Breath.

When you begin your yoga practice, you often start by standing in Mountain Pose. Standing in stillness and silence allows for the opportunity to focus on the ujjayi breathing. Let's practice this exercise, though, while seated in Easy Pose. Sit up nice and tall with an extended spine and straight back. Close your eyes to begin your journey inward. In your stillness, simply be aware that you are breathing. Breathe in and out through your nose. You don't have to do anything special with the breath at this point. Just be aware that you are breathing. You may feel breath move in and out of your body...perhaps through your nostrils.

From here you will shift that sensation of nostril breathing to throat breathing. This will help to engage the ujjayi breath. To initiate the throat breathing, allow your mouth to open wide and take a few breaths in and out through your mouth. As you draw in breath, feel the airy hollowness of breath moving into the back of your mouth. You may even feel a coolness hit the back your throat. As you exhale, breathe out as if you are fogging a mirror. (Place your hand in front of your mouth to mimic a mirror to simulate this exercise. Feel the warm air hit your hand as you release the breath.) Do that a few times then continue this process of breathing with your mouth CLOSED. You may feel that same sensation in the back of your throat as you did when you had your mouth open. You've begun ujjayi breathing.

If you you continue this practice, you may find that you can take slower and deeper breaths. Also, you may hear a sound which we sometimes refer to as the Ujjayi Sound. It may sound like an ocean wave rolling onto the beach. As you deepen the breath here, really feel the expansion of your lungs. You may feel your chest rise with each inhale. As you exhale, try to maintain the victorious breath high in your chest by engaging your abdominal muscles. Feel your navel draw in toward your spine. This is the abdominal lock or Uddiyana Bandha. Again, the more you practice this style of breath, you will also expand the capacity of your lungs AND strengthen your core.

Taking deep breaths is an intention process and takes your full attention to do so. Further, Ujjayi Breathing helps to calm the circulatory system so it can help relieve stress and anxiety. Practice Ujjayi Breath for about

2 minutes and experience the calming effects of the practice. When you are in your next yoga class, be sure to connect to this way of breathing to help guide you and move you through your practice.

4.
SELF CARE

"It's not selfish to love yourself, take care of yourself, and to make your happiness a priority. It's necessary." - Mandy Hale

In this section, we will focus on taking care of yourself. This is a very important idea that we all need to practice more often. We walk through our lives doing many things for others. If you're a parent, for example, you tend to the care for your children. In order for us to be effective caretakers, we must first take good care of ourselves.

1. Slow Down
2. A Sigh of Relief
3. Concentration
4. Inner Strength
5. Rest

1. Slow Down

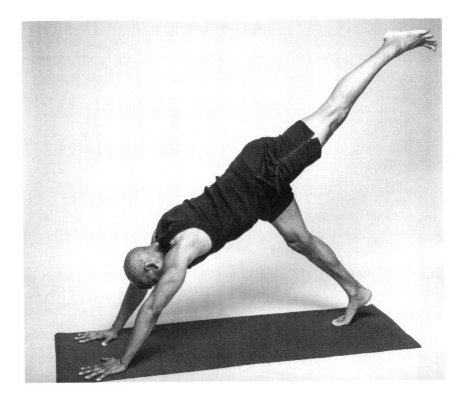

Featured Pose:
Sun Salutations, Ujjayi Breath

As we get older, it seems that we have MORE to do with LESS time. (How did that happen?) We constantly try to cram too many things to do in our already business schedules. Often, we run out of time, and the daily list is rarely completed; more items just seem to be added to the never-ending list.

"If only there were more hours in the day," we say to ourselves. "If only I could move faster to get all of these things done."

Why not do the opposite? Appreciate the number of hours you have in the day and actually move slower to complete your to-do list. You might find that by taking the time to slow down, your mind is clearer, more rational, and can make logical decisions that lead to successful completions rather than running around constantly worrying rather than doing.

In this yoga practice, try moving through a simple Sun Salutation slower than you usually move. The idea is to move with a slower pace of breath. Start by standing in Mountain Pose and become aware of the sensation of breath. Once you have made this breath connection, begin an engaging series of Ujjayi Breaths to bring yourself to greater awareness of each inhale and exhale. (If you've forgotten how to do Ujjayi breathing, please refer to Section 1: Awareness, Chapter 1: Awareness & Breath.)

Continue to stand still and silent in Mountain Pose engaged in the breath and begin to pay attention to the pace of each inhale and the pace of each exhale. Breathe in a fashion where the pace of the exhale matches the pace of the inhale. Now, count the beats associated with the pace of the inhale and the pace of the exhale. For example, when you draw in one breath, you might find that it takes 3 beats. (Try counting slowly, like this...."one –Mississippi, two-Mississippi, etc.)

Once you have taken note of the pace of each breath, try slowing down the pace of the inhale and exhale so the rate is now 4 beats rather than 3. Try doing this two more times until the pace of your breathing effort has slowed down significantly. Now it is time to move. Still using this new pace of breath, begin your Sun Salutation. Each movement now coincides with the pace and rhythm of the Ujjayi Breath. You'll find that you'll move through your practice much slower.

Sun Salutation: Series A
Mountain Pose
Forward Fold
Plank
Chaturanga Dandasana
Upward Facing Dog
Downward Facing Dog
Forward Fold
Mountain Pose

The intention is to practice moving slower through the course of your day. Pace yourself. Take your time. You may find that you are more calm and collected and able to get more done in your busy day.

2. A Sigh of Relief

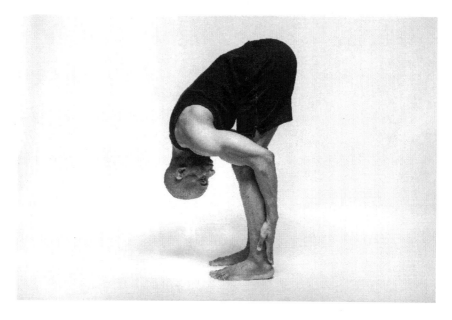

Featured Pose:
Uttanasana (Standing Forward Fold)

Have you ever encountered a challenge in your life, but then felt relieved after you successfully overcame the challenge? What is one of the first things you did? Perhaps experienced a big sigh of relief, right?

What happens within your body when you sigh? Typically we have held some sort of tension in the body then when you breathe out, usually through the mouth, that tension is released. You may even make a sound: an audible sign indicating that the tension is no longer in your body. One may feel a sense of lightness, a weight completed lifted.

Sometimes in a yoga practice, in order to move deeper into a pose, it may be necessary to experience that audible sigh of relief. Try this breathing sensation with the following yoga sequence.

Start by standing in Mountain Pose. Begin your Ujjayi Breathing. Remember, this flow of breath is typically through the nose; your mouth is closed. You will feel the dynamic breath move in and out of your nostrils, but the effort of the breath comes from the muscles in the back of your throat. Once you feel a greater connection to the breath, begin your Sun Salutation. Complete a Series A (3 times through) to bring warmth and opening to the body.

Sun Salutation: Series A
Mountain Pose
Forward Fold
Plank
Chaturanga Dandasana
Upward Facing Dog
Downward Facing Dog
Forward Fold
Mountain Pose

After you have completed your warm up, return to the Forward Fold Posture. It is perfectly fine to be in this pose with bent knees. (There is no rule that says you have to be in a Forward Fold with straight legs!) In order to experience more release and straighter legs (if that is your intention) then you can use your dynamic breath – and a sigh of relief – to help you achieve that goal.

While in your Forward Fold, hold onto each elbow or the backs of your legs. This will create more weight in the body allowing you to go deeper into the pose. Pay attention to your breathing: breathe in through your nose, then, with a sigh, breathe out through your mouth. See if your body went deeper into the pose.

You can continue to move deeper by doing the following: allow your hips to lift a little higher toward the ceiling while at the same time feel the backs of your knees move toward the back of the room. These do not have to be big movements. Move gently and carefully into the depth of your posture. Don't forget to sigh.

Physically, over time, this will create more length and flexibility in your hamstrings. Emotionally and mentally, think of this exercise as a way to experience release of tension; as a way to create more space in your heart and mind so you can move forward on your life journey.

3. Concentration

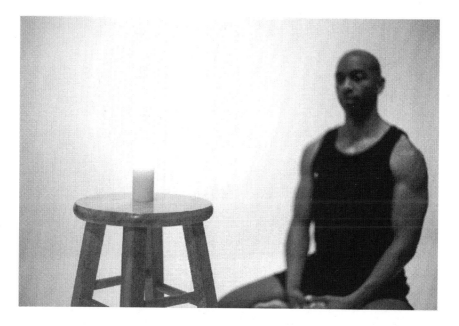

<u>Featured Pose:</u>
Candle Gazing

<u>Recommended Reading:</u>
The Yoga Sutras

The Yoga Sutras, written around the 2nd century by Patanjali, is an attempt to define and standardize Classical Yoga. It is composed of 196 sutras (sutra = thread) that read as verses and forms the structural framework of the yoga practice. The Yoga Sutra is an eight-limbed (Astanga) path that leads one to completeness; a path that leads to the connectivity to the divine.

In the third chapter of the Yoga Sutras, Patanjali writes about Supernatural Abilities and Gifts (Vibhuti Pada). The verses begin with the importance of meditation as a particular limb that brings one to the connection to the divine:

III, 1
Contemplation
is
the confining
of thought
to one point.

III, 2
Meditation
depends upon this
foundation for directing thoughts
into a continuous flow
of awareness.

To practice this method of meditation, I want to introduce the practice of Candle Gazing. I have taught this simple method of meditation in several yoga classes and my students have been amazed at the results they received. One mentioned, "I let go of some old emotional baggage...the candle triggered something and I started to let go of old issues." Candle Gazing (Trataka) is an ancient Indian practice that is said to help focus the mind, improve concentration, and is very calming.

Here's how it is done:
Light a candle and place it on a low table. Sit on the floor in a comfortable meditation posture (like Half Lotus or Easy Pose). The candle flame should be at eye-level while you're seated. If you are new to this practice, you will start your candle gazing at 30 seconds per round. As you grow more accustomed to the practice, you can extend the time you gaze at the flame.

To begin, stare at the candle flame for 30 seconds without blinking. (Although you cannot look at a clock, just get a sense of how long 30 seconds is.) You may have the urge to blink or your focus may become blurred during the exercise. Whatever happens, keep your attention on the flame. After 30 seconds, close your eyes for an additional 30 seconds. An after-image of the flame may still be present in your mind's eye. Focus on this "internal flame." After about 30 seconds, repeat the candle gazing. Do this for at least 3 rounds. At the end of your last round, place your cupped palms over your eyes and let the eyes relax in this new darkness. This is called palming.

This exercise can be done with any inanimate object and be done just about anywhere. (Try doing it at your desk and stare at the tip of a pencil.) The idea is to focus your vision and your mind. The result is a sense of calm and relaxation. Try it when you're under stress. Better yet, include it in your regular morning daily routine to start your day. You may find that you have a sense of calm throughout the entire day.

4. Inner Strength

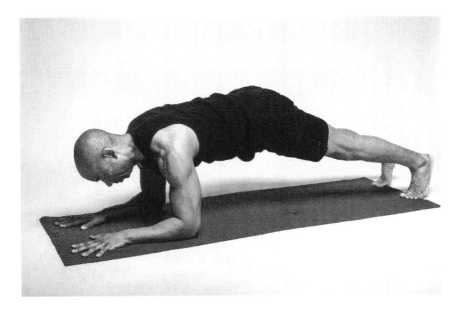

Featured Pose:
Makara Adho Mukha Svanasana (Dolphin Plank Pose)

Sometimes we can experience a lack of strength in some life situations. You feel like you couldn't manage a difficult job at work, you didn't feel you had the strength to help a friend in need, or it may be you just couldn't push that heavy weight at the gym this morning. Whatever it is, sometimes we would like to feel stronger. Often, too, we look for strength from the outside....someone or something else is going to give us the strength that we need or desire.

You go to your clergy person to seek guidance; you read about a new device or technology that will improve your memory; you try a new supplement that will give you more energy in the day. All of these are external ways to improve strength AND they can be very effective. One thing to remember, though, is that strength can come from within. YOU have the power and strength within YOU to achieve better direction, memory, or health. Believe in yourself and the power comes.

The pose for your home yoga practice is a modification of plank pose. You will do it on your forearms (Dolphin Plank Pose) which brings more attention to your abdominal muscles. Often when we focus on core strength, we think of our abdominal muscles. A reminder that your core incorporates the entire trunk of your body. In yoga we often focus on the low back and abdominal muscles. This is one such pose.

Start by coming to your hands and knees on your yoga mat. Gently lower yourself so that you are on your forearms and on your toes. Create a strong straight line with the entire body. (If you need to, it's ok to lower your knees to the floor, but keep your core body engaged.) Be aware if your low back is sinking or if your rear is lifted too high in the air. Create a sturdy table-top-like posture. This will involve engaging your core muscles. Do so by tilting your pelvis AND feel your belly button pull up to your spine. This will be easy to do when you focus on your exhales. When you release the breath, also feel the tilting of the pelvis and the navel pulling upward toward your spine. Here, you are engaging an abdominal lock so you can feel solid in your pose. Also, feel the forearms hug together as if you were a squeezing a ball between them. This is how you experience inner strength: hug toward your center.

I tell my students that when you hug/hold inward, you create more strength inside of you. Imagine a person climbing up a pole. The tighter they hold on, the longer they will remain on the pole and perhaps the higher they can climb. Once they loosen that grip, they fall. Holding this plank pose can be the same; be sure to feel a sensation of hugging in toward your mid-line: your spine. Hold this pose as long as you can. If you happen to have a timer, 30 seconds to 1 minute would be quite effective. Or take 10-20 breaths. Afterward, come to Child's Pose to relax the entire body. Here, remind yourself of the strength that you hold within you. You'll find that you can climb higher and reach all of your goals.

5. Rest

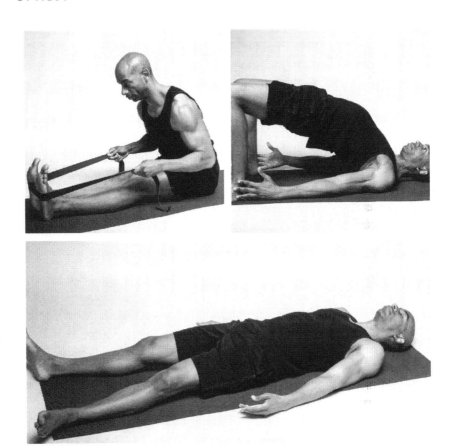

Featured Poses:
Urdhva Dhanurasana (Wheel Pose) or Setu Bandha Sarvangasana
(Bridge Pose)
Paschimottanasana (Seated Forward Fold)
Savasana (Corpse Pose)

Recommended Reading:
"The Heart of Yoga" by T.K.V. Desikachar

Ever find yourself moving throughout your busy day without taking a moment to rest? You wake up one morning, knowing you have a busy schedule, and the moment your feet hit the floor from the bed, you're off and running. Typically it's non-stop: get the kids to school, go to work, attend business meetings, a yoga class at noon, more meetings, more deadlines to complete, take the kids to soccer, go grocery shopping, pick up the kids, cook dinner, clean the kitchen, prepare tomorrow's lunches, and MAYBE sit for 30 minutes to catch the evening news. Before you know it, it's 10:30 and you're in bed only to find that you have to get up the next day and do it all over again.

It seems the only time we allow ourselves to rest is when we go to sleep. You've been constantly moving for 15 hours and you only give yourself 6, MAYBE 8 hours of sleep. Are you providing your body and mind enough down-time to recuperate? This home practice reminds us that it is very important to take intentional rest time throughout our busy days.

T.K.V. Desikachar, in "The Heart of Yoga" reminds us to take a much needed rest during dynamic yoga practices and even between poses. "There is no rule to follow regarding rest," he says. "...if we need a rest, we take one." An example is to move into a dynamic posture like an intense backbend (dhanurasana) then into a counter pose like a seated forward fold (paschimottanasana).

Wheel Pose / Bridge Pose
Start by lying on your back with your knees bent. Be sure your knees and feet are about hip-distance apart. Your heels should be relatively close to your backside. If you plan to move into a full backbend, Wheel Pose, place your hands up near your shoulders with your fingertips pointing toward your shoulders. If you plan to move into Bridge Pose, simple place your arms along the sides of your body on the floor.

With an intentional exhale, press your lower back into the floor. This will tilt the pelvis and engage your core to support your backbend. With your next exhale, lift your hips into the sky. If you're moving into Wheel Pose, press your hands firmly into the floor with your elbows hugging closely to your head and lift your upper body off the floor until you are in a full backbend. If moving into Bridge Pose, lift the hips on the exhale then squeeze your shoulder blades together underneath you to help support the pose. Hold your backbend for 1 minute or 10-20 breaths.

Slowly and carefully lower yourself down to the floor when you have completed your breaths in the backbend. Lie flat on the floor in Savasana for another 30 seconds to 1 minute. Afterward, draw your knees in toward your chest and gently rock yourself up to a seated posture.

Seated Forward Fold
Extend your legs straight out in front of you and sit up nice and tall. Extend your arms overhead with an inhale and on your exhale, while hinging from your hips, fold forward bringing your heart closer to your legs. If you're able, reach out and touch your toes. If you are unable to reach your feet, simply rest your hands anywhere on your legs. Hold this pose for 1 minute or 10-20 breaths.

Both of these poses can be intense, but are counter poses to one another. If you start with a forward fold in your home practice, finish with a backbend to help counteract the intensity. More importantly, be sure to rest in between each intense posture. Lying in Savasana (Corpse Pose) is a perfect relaxing posture.

Use this home practice as a reminder that it is important to take intentional rests throughout the day to help counteract the intensity of your busy schedule. For example, before you get out of the car to step into the grocery store, sit in your car for a minute with your eyes closed and focus on your breathing. After sitting at your computer for several hours, stand up and stretch the entire body (perhaps Extended Mountain Pose) to help counter the sitting sensation. Instead of watching the evening news, take a few minutes to practice Candle Gazing (Section 4, Chapter 3).

There are many things we can do to counteract the wear and tear of our busy lives. Sometimes it just takes a minute or two to give yourself the gift of restfulness.

5.
HONORING SELF

"Humble yourself, and you shall be honored. Honor yourself, and you shall be humbled." - Unknown

The final section of this book focuses on honoring yourself. You are the most important element if you are to be effective in the world you live in. Your doings with family members, co-workers, friends, and community can only be worthwhile and successful if you first cherish and honor who and what you are.

1. Be Kind To Yourself
2. Be A Warrior: Part 1
3. Be A Warrior: Part 2
4. Be A Warrior: Part 3
5. Sit In Your Perfect

1. Be Kind To Yourself

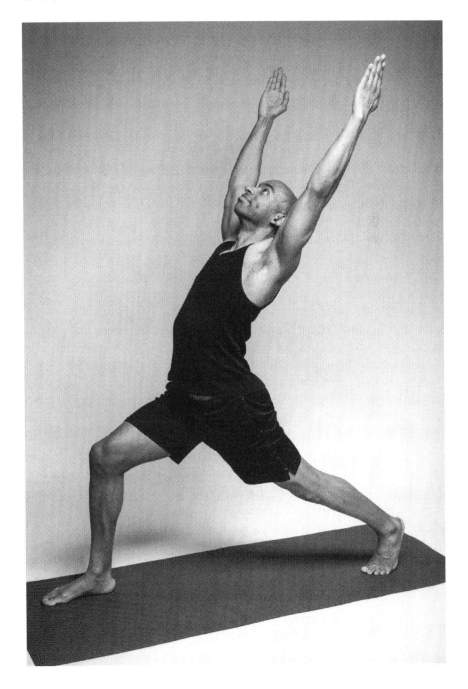

Featured Pose:
Alasana (High Lunge or Cresent Moon)

Recommended Reading:
"The Yamas & Niyamas: Exploring Yoga's Ethical Practice" by Deborah Adele

The Yamasa and Niyamas are yoga's ten ethical guidelines which are thought of as the foundation for skillful living. The first ethical guideline is called Ahimsa (uh-HIM-saw) which means non-violence. Ahimsa is the first of five restraints (Yamas) yogis are encouraged to practice. Ahimsa is the awareness and practice of non-violence in thought, speech, and action. It promotes the practices of compassion, love, understanding, patience, self-love, and worthiness. I particularly like the aspect of self-love, gentleness, and kindness toward yourself. When practiced within, they eventually become an outward expression of self toward others.

As we move from pose to pose in a vinyasa flow, we can move slowly with intention and attention. The idea is to be fully aware of the postures you are in, as well as take your time to move deeper (as the body is able) into any particular pose. If we simply take our time as we progress deeper into our physical bodies, the body will, in turn, respond kindly.

For example, if you are in a lunging posture (i.e. Cresent Moon Pose or Alasana), you can move deeper into the pose one breath at a time. As you inhale, fully extend the rear leg back by pushing the heel towards the floor and extend the arms higher into the air. On the exhale, bend the forward knee more (only by 1/2 an inch) to move deeper into the pose.

When we push our bodies by moving too quickly, forcefully, or without intention, this is a shock to the physical self which may result in injury or pain. If you are looking for greater flexibility and you want to maintain flexibility, the slower you go, the better and long lasting the results. Move too fast, and the body reacts rather than responds and flexibility is not attained or it is only temporary.

You can do this with any yoga posture. Practice slowly with intention and attention which translates to being more kind (non-violent) to yourself. You are practicing Ahimsa. This principle, of course, works off the mat, too. When you carry negative self thoughts or put yourself down, you are practicing Himsa or violence toward yourself.

To read more about yoga principles and philosophy, a good place to start is understanding the Yamas (restraints) and Niyamas (observances). They are the first two limbs of the Eight Limbs of Yoga. Together, they are ten guidelines for leading a healthier and happier lifestyle. They bring spiritual awareness into a social context.

2. Be A Warrior – Part 1

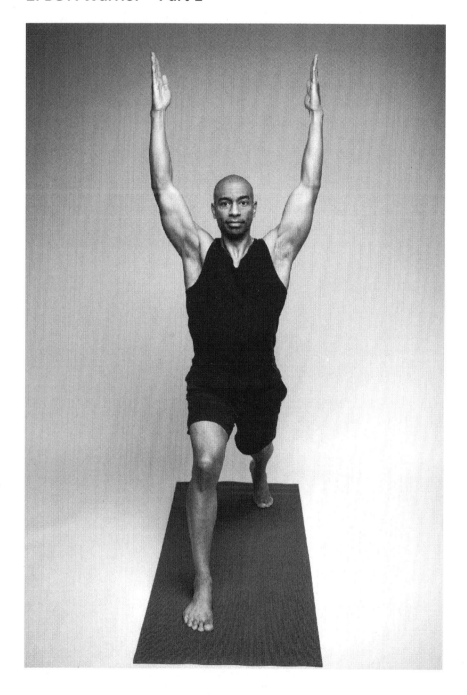

Featured Pose:
Virabhadrasana I (Warrior I Pose)

For the next three chapters, we will focus on the three variations of Virabhadrasana (Warrior Pose). In Sanskrit, the word "vira" means "hero." Virabhadra is a hero warrior from Hindu mythology. He is said to have a thousand arms and was created by the Lord Shiva to avenge his wife Sati. Like many Hindu stories, they are metaphors that can relate to our everyday lives. The idea of Virabhadra is a reminder that we are the warriors and conquerers of our own weaknesses. By nurturing our inner warrior, we prepare ourselves to deal with our own life challenges.

Here is the story of Virabhdra. Daksha, Sati's father, didn't approve of Sati's marriage to Shiva, so when Daksha decided to host a sacrificial festival, he didn't invite Shiva or Sati, even though the other Hindu gods were invited. Sati was hurt by this, but decided to go to the festival to confront Daksha.

Daksha asked why Sati was there since she wasn't invited. He snidely asked if she had finally come to her senses and left that "wild animal of a husband". Sati was saddened and humiliated, and decided to end her own life, not wanting to be associated with her father anymore. In one version of this story she throws herself into the sacrificial fires, and in another version she goes into a meditative state to increase her own inner fire, and her body bursts into flame.

When Shiva heard the news of his wife's death, he was first devastated, then enraged. From the locks of hair that he tore out in his fury, he created Virabhadra. (Other versions say Virabhadra sprung up from where Shiva's matted locks of hair hit the ground, or that he arose from drops of Shiva's sweat during his fury.)

Virabhadra was huge and terrible -- he had a thousand arms, three burning eyes and fiery hair, and he wore a garland of skulls.

Shiva ordered Virabhadra, the "auspicious hero", (vira = hero, bhadra = auspicious) to kill all the guests at the sacrificial festival, including the other gods. Virabhadra did this, and also cut off Daksha's head. But when Shiva saw the bloody aftermath of this battle, his anger left him and he felt remorse. The slain gods were miraculously healed, and Shiva replaced Daksha's head with a goat's head. Daksha and the other gods honored Shiva for this, calling him "Shankar", the "kind and benevolent one."

Warrior I:
The Warrior I Pose is a lunging posture. Start with your right foot at the top of your mat with your bent knee (about 90 degrees) and toes pointing directly forward. Your left leg is straight and your foot is near the back edge of your mat. Be sure the entire foot is on the floor and it may be turned at a comfortable angle so that the back edge of your foot meets the floor. Your torso is facing forward and your arms are reaching straight up toward the sky.

Warrior I opens the chest and lungs, allowing for better breathing. It also creates more flexibility in the shoulders, back, and hips. You will find that this a great hip and hip flexor opener. Further, it strengthens the legs. This is a good pose to prepare for back-bending poses.

The image of the arms shooting skyward represents Virabhadra emerging from the earth as he comes to life. Metaphorically, we can use this image of the arising warrior as the preparation for the battles and challenges ahead. It is the decision to take charge and move forward to face your life obstacles. While in Virabhdrasana I, bring to mind any challenges that you are NOW ready to face and conquer. With each breath, conjure up your Inner Warrior. (Repeat the pose on the other side.)

3. Be A Warrior – Part 2

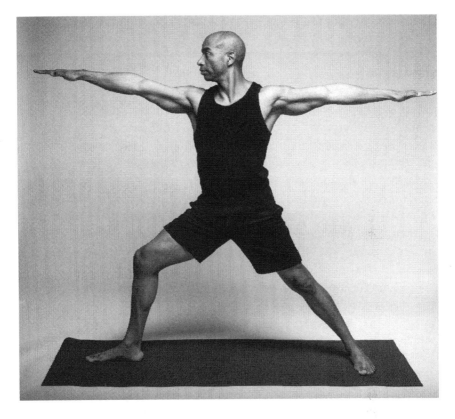

Featured Pose:
Virabhadrasana II (Warrior II Pose)

In the story of Virabhadra, we recall that he came to life from the locks of Shiva's hair. In the Virabhadrasana I Pose where the arms are extended overhead, we are reminded of how this warrior sprung to life. The symbol of this great Hindu warrior is that we can be in a position to face our own obstacles and challenges.

What challenges have you faced this week? Relationship? Illness? Work stress? Car troubles? Even in the face of these obstacles, have you felt at the ready to deal and manage these obstacles? Warrior I had you poised and ready for these life events. Now it is time to take action.

The story states that Shiva ordered Virabhadra to kill all the guests at the sacrificial festival, including the other gods. Virabhadra did this. Yes, this is a gory depiction, but a reminder that sometimes facing our challenges may not always be an easy task to do. We find the warrior within and move forward.

Warrior II
In this yoga pose, our arms are extended outward - they are parallel to the earth. The extended arms represent the thousand arms of Virabhadra. Our drishti, or focus, is over the front arm. (If your left foot is forward, then your focus is over the left hand.)

Come into Virabhadrasana II. Refer to the previous chapter on how to position your feet and legs. Feel rooted and connected into the earth with both feet. Be sure your front knee is stacked directly over your ankle to allow for proper and healthy structure of the pose as well as protection of your knee joint. Your torso remains upright and proud.

As you hold this pose (5-10 breaths), take your gaze forward over your extended arm. This aspect of the Warrior Pose represents Virabhadra as he sights Daksha at the festival, readying himself to slay Daksha, a metaphor for slaying our own ignorance and ego. See yourself standing in this warrior-confidence moving forward to conquer your battles. Be sure to repeat this posture on both sides.

4. Be A Warrior – Part 3

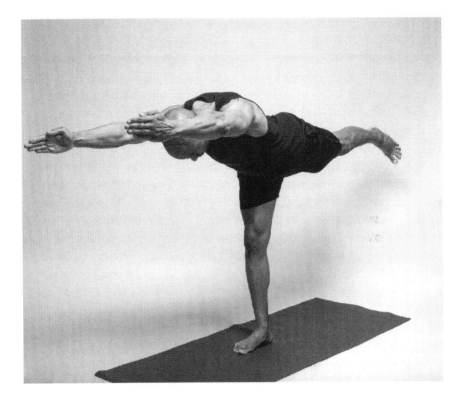

Featured Pose:
Virabhadrasana III (Warrior III Pose)

"Establishing his arrival for all to see, Virabhadra then sites his
opponent, Daksha. Moving swiftly and precisely, he takes his sword and
cuts off Daksha's head."

This passage illustrates the progression of the Hindu Warrior as he sets
site on this opponent and moves in for the kill. It is the transition from
Warrior II to Warrior III.

Virabhdrasana III is often considered the most challenging of the
Warrior poses. It allows us to strengthen the abdominal muscles as well
as improves our posture. It brings better balance and greater stamina,
not only in our practice, but also in our lives.

Warrior III is slightly different from the first two Warrior poses since you are balancing on one foot rather than feeling solid with both feet on the ground. While standing on the right foot, the rest of the body is perpendicular to the floor with both arms extended out in front of you (visualize flying through the sky like Superman). Your left leg is extended out behind you, also parallel to the floor. The aspect of this pose represents Virabhadra as he drives forward to slay Daksha. It further represents the yoga practitioner slaying the ego or the obstacles and challenges that need to be conquered.

As you move into this posture on the first side, start by feeling very rooted into the ground with your standing leg. The energy from the balance comes from your core; your abdominals are fully engaged and tight. Energy for the rest of the pose comes from your core center. The right foot drives strongly into the floor, but the strength comes from the top of the leg - the hip and hip flexor. Your core strength also helps to extend both arms forward. (As a modification, do this pose in front of a wall. Your hands or fingertips can touch the wall as a way to help manage the balance of the pose.)

Further, the left leg is extended straight out back behind you. The glutes and hamstrings are fully engaged to help with the lifting of the leg so it remains parallel with the floor. (Likewise, as a modification, you can face away from a wall in the pose. The toes or foot of the extended leg can touch the wall to help maintain the balance.) Hold the pose for at least 5 breaths then repeat it on the other side.

Remember, while holding this posture, bring to mind the obstacles and challenges you have been facing in recent weeks. Now is the time to take action. You realize, now, that these challenges no longer serve you in your life and you are ready to break down these walls. Movement and action come from your center - your core - your third chakra. While in the pose, imagine you are in flight - flying forward to face and remove your fears. Believe in the strength you possess as you step forth, like the bold Hindu Warrior, and conquer your obstacles.

5. Sit In Your Perfect

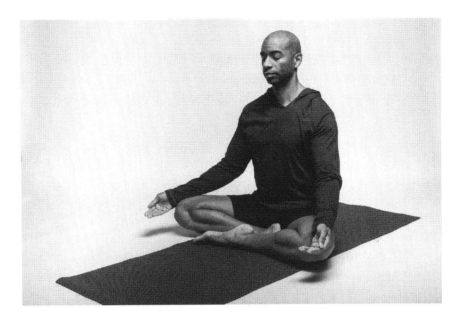

Featured Pose:
Siddhasana (Perfect Pose)

Take a look in the mirror. Do you like what you see? I hope you do. You are beautiful. You are handsome. You are amazing! Do those words sound foreign to you? They shouldn't! Because they are true.

Sometimes we look at ourselves and become our own worst critics: I'm overweight. I have blotchy skin. I'm too short. My hair is going gray. (Shall I go on?)

We forget about the beauty that we possess inside and out. We forget that we are only human beings....living a human experience, capable of making mistakes, but also capable of accomplishing great things. We sometimes forget about our gifts, traits, and talents: I'm organized. I can play the flute. I can make a mean pumpkin pie!

In spite of our perceived flaws....we are perfect. YOU are PERFECT! You are the way you are supposed to be. Media likes to tell us differently;

we need to be someone or something else. Turn off the television!

Let's take a moment in our yoga practice today to remember the reality of your perfection.

Take a seat on the floor. You will move into what is called Perfect Pose. It's like sitting in a cross-legged position, but you will place one leg in front of the other or stack one leg on top of the other rather than interlacing the legs.

The Sanskrit word for Perfect Pose is Siddhasana. Siddha means Semi-Devine Being with Great Sanctity. The posture gets its name because the person performing the pose attempts to emulate a sage who is perfect or a prophet who is accomplished. (That sounds just like YOU.)

This pose is suitable for a seated meditation which is what you'll do for your home yoga practice. As you sit in Perfect Pose, begin your deep yoga breath to bring awareness and focus to your inner self. Call to mind all your positive traits, talents, and qualities. Name the things you like and love about yourself. Even bring to mind events or circumstances in your life that made you proud and smile (e.g. job promotion, graduation.) Sit in your perfection. If negative thoughts, ideas, or beliefs enter your consciousness, take a deep Ujjayi breath to clear that thought from your Being. That is NOT your TRUE SELF. Only bring to mind those positive aspects and features of yourself. Remain here for 3-5 minutes.

After this practice, return to the mirror and say THREE POSITIVE things about yourself OUTLOUD. Then smile.

PROLOGUE
Continue The Journey

Now that you have come to the end of this book, know that this is not the end. This is only the beginning of your journey. Hopefully, the elements in this book have fostered some awareness that has deepened your connection to Self and the taking care of Self. The journey is continuous. We often find ourselves in circumstances when we need a little more strength, more clarity, more guidance. Return to this book to help you with that guidance forward. Feel free to carry this book around like a handy guide. When you need a little inspiration for a home practice or a quick pick-me-up, turn to any page of this guide and practice the intention. Continue your journey. Witness yourself grow and prosper as you bring deeper meaning to your yoga practice and apply it to your everyday life events. Namaste.

ABOUT THE AUTHOR

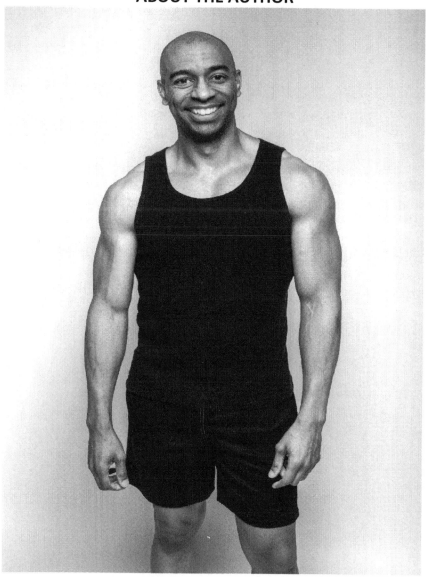

John Cottrell is originally from Oakland, California and is now residing in Salt Lake City, Utah. John is formally educated in clinical psychology having earned a Bachelor of Science degree from Santa Clara University and a Master of Science degree and Ph.D. from Pacific Graduate School of Psychology in Palo Alto.

John moved to Salt Lake City in 1994 for his clinical psychology internship with Valley Mental Health. There he gained a broad range of experience including: child and adolescent psychotherapy, drug and alcohol treatment, psychological and neuropsychological testing, and group/couples therapy.

John has always been fascinated with fitness and became devoted to this lifestyle in 1999. While still working as a psychotherapist, John taught fitness classes ranging from weight lifting to hip hop dance aerobics in the gym. John added yoga to his fitness routine in 2000. He has been able to use his education in psychology and devotion to fitness and yoga to understand and offer the benefits of a body and mind connection.

As a certified yoga instructor (RYT 500), personal trainer, and sports nutritionist, John offers a variety of ways to create healthy living. He now teaches a variety of yoga classes in the greater Salt Lake City area. He is also on the faculty of Inbody Yoga Academy in Salt Lake where he provides training to those seeking certification in yoga therapy. John started his own business, mbody in 2008 and offers Yoga Life Coaching, Nutrition Coaching, Personal Training, private and group yoga lessons, workshops, and retreats. He launched a men's yoga clothing line, *mbody men's yoga clothing*, in 2012.

Made in the USA
San Bernardino, CA
09 June 2016